Essential Oils Collection:

100 Best Recipes For All Occasions + Holistic

Remedies That Really Work

Table of content:

Book 3

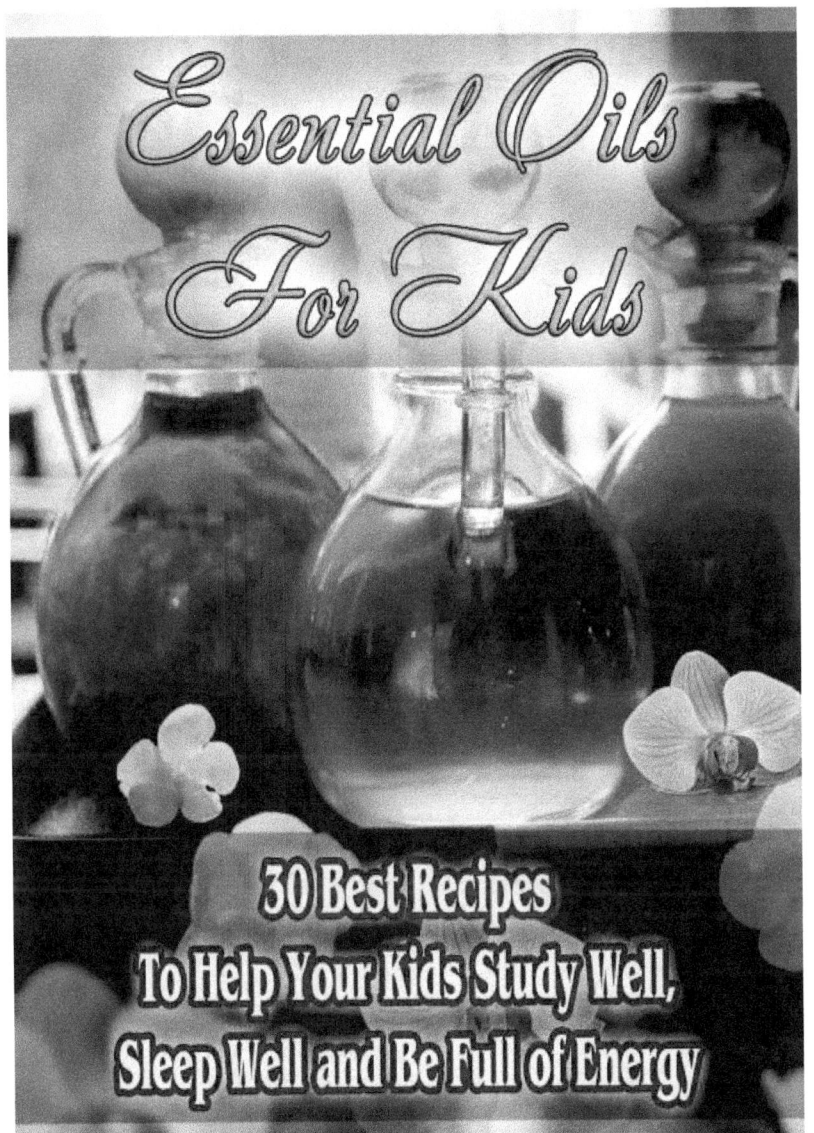

Essential Oils For Kids

30 Best Recipes To Help Your Kids Study Well, Sleep Well and Be Full of Energy

Lora Brexner

Essential Oils for Kids:

30 Best Recipes to Help Your Kids Study Well, Sleep Well and Be Full of Energy

Introduction

Many parents get concerned when it comes to trying something with their kids. They think that it might suit them according to their age but that is not the case with essential oils blend. Essential oils are natural and they heal no matter what your age is. It can be used on the toddlers, infants, kids, adults or any person. They only give positive results whoever uses it and never works against it. You just need to know the right blend and if your child likes it fragrance then you can keep on using it to heal them.

Mostly the toddlers give hard time to the parents so you can use the recipes for them to calm them. Moms do not get time to do the house chores due to which they feel angry and scold their children. You can use these recipes and stay calm by yourself and keep your children calm as well.

The essential oils recipes will help you get rid of crankiness and you will feel relaxed that your kid is playing without disturbing you. You can spend time with your spouse easily when your child is sleeping calmly because of the essential oil massage.

You will see the difference in the environment, as well as the behavior of your kid. Many practitioners use essential oils as a therapy for their patients because of the natural herbs included in it. Anything which is natural will never harm you so get started with the perfect blend recipes of diffusers which can make your house smell beautiful and keep your kids aligned with normal activities with staying calm and easy.

Essential Oils for Kids Health

Essential oils do not have any side or hidden effects. You will be glad to use the oils on your kids because they provide ultimate relief which you may be having a long time. They are natural and do not harm you at all. You only need to know the right blends for the specific thing, and you will see how it heals you perfectly without even knowing it.

Essential oils have played a dynamic role in the history where it used to be set as an example to heal someone through the natural means. The essential oils are extracted from the aroma plants which is why the smell of it is so soothing that you wish to keep on smelling it forever.

Some people have aromas of essential oils in their home to feel better, and it also enhances the mood due to which they have diffusers at home. Here are some of the factors which will make you realize the important of essential oils.

- **Treats Minor Illness for the Kids**

Many people have allergies or some illnesses prolong which becomes a tension for you already. It diffuses the basic illness which you can get on daily routines such as flu, coughing and all. The vapors in the air have the power to make you feel better on your chest and head.

Once you inhale it naturally just like you breathe in the air, it will make you feel okay. You will forget that you have the flu and it will stop. It is only the game of the brain. Once that part is normal, you will normally be functioning too, but if that part is a mess, then there is no way out for you to escape it.

- **Creativity Emerges**

When your brain cells are charged, you are active and working more intelligently, but when you get tired, it gets hard to comprehend anything because of the low functionality.

You can escape such situations by having the essential oils at home. It will make your brain function fast all the time whether you are tired or not. You will be able to focus on the thing which you are working on even if you are tired.

There are some of the oils which help you gain the energy and keep your muscles active. If you use the essential oils regularly, there will be a clear difference between the before and after situation.

- **Brings Calmness to the Kids**

Staying calm sometimes becomes hard, but the essential oil does so. It keeps the kids calm even in the situation where there is a mess, and you can get angry. Sometimes when we are frustrated, we tend to take it out of our friends and family, but with the help of having the essential oils and the beautiful scents around you, you will be calmer than before.

- **Cost –Effective**

Essential oil saves you from a lot of the things which can occur to you if you do not have it. It saves you money, and it is a one-time cost which you will have to bear.

You won't have to pay visits to the doctor because the prior job of the essential oils is to keep you healthy psychologically and physically. That is what it takes if you have just one essential oil and perfect recipes of essential oil to be poured into it.

- **No Mood Swings for Children**

Improving moods is the top most response of the essential oils. They work like magic on kids' mood no matter if they are angry or irritate, it works like anything on them.

It turns the negative emotions into positive ones naturally. You can make the positive environment if your brain is working towards that direction too. You can be a hope to someone as well who is depressed from life. Take out time for your spouse with having the essential oils at home, and you will see how the atmosphere turns romantic like nothing before.

- **Relief of Minor Pains**

When we feel pain anywhere, we tend to panic more than the pain. It is because our brain does not accept that something has happened to the body and we tend to fall weak in a trap of getting emotional.

We lose our mind due to which it gets on our head and tension increases the pain by keeping the muscles stressed. You can also use some of the essential oils as a massage which will heal your muscles of the kids. For a headache, just apply the necessary essential oil, and the scent of it will make you feel better for sure.

- **Sleep Peacefully With Essential Oil Blend**

We all know that if you do not get enough sleep time, then your brain activity tends to slow down over the period no matter how hard you try to stay up. It is beyond a human's capacity to stay up for more than 48 hours continuously.

When you have had a hard day, that is when the essential oil works the best for you. It keeps you calm and makes you sleep within seconds with a deep night sleep. Even if you get like 5 hours of sleep daily and that too deep, it will be enough for you to carry on with the tough days. If you feel like taking the essential oils to your office, you can do that too, and the environment will be so friendly which you will love.

Your kid will love to wake up for school every day because of having such a comfortable environment. Human brains are complicated which is why there are so many problems in the world which cannot be resolved and keeps on exaggerating. Well, get a good night sleep with the application of essential oils, and once you get a hold of it, then it is hard to stop it.

- **Breathing Gets Normal**

If you are someone whose chest gets congested every other day, then the essential oil is best for you. The allergies get eliminate with making you breathe faster and easier than before. You won't be breathing fast once you have inhaled the scents of essential oil or while climbing the stairs too.

Keep the essential oils in your room, and you will see the difference that you do not tend to breathe heavier anymore. Heavy breathing can be dangerous because it indicates a lot of weakness in you. You need to make sure to check with the doctor if it does not fix with the essential oils.

Chapter 1 – Energetic Blends for Your School Going Children

A lot of people go through a lot of problems with their children nowadays without them knowing about it and they get irritated for no reason. There are many causes due to which you can feel tired such as stress, fatigue, hormones, constipation, low sugar level, poor posture, food and much more.

Kids go to school every day and then end up having pains by night. Sometimes you do not get to know which way to go and what to do to get some relief which is why you start giving the medications which are not so recommended for the kids.

You can try the awesome recipes for the school going child who will wake up fresh and stay happy all the time. It is necessary that the kids have their moods happy because then it turns into a frustration and becomes a bad signs for their future. Check out the amazing fragrance blends which can keep your child fresh and going with the daily routine life.

Recipe 01: Roll-On Blend – Sweet Dreams

Ingredients:

- 10 ml roller bottle: 1
- Coconut oil: 2 Teaspoons
- Roman Chamomile Essential Oil: 1 Drop
- Geranium Essential Oil: 1 Drop
- Waterproof Label: 1

Directions:

Add essential oils with coconut oil in the roller bottle. Afterwards, put inside the roller attachment along with its lid. Place the waterproof label and keep away at a safe place.

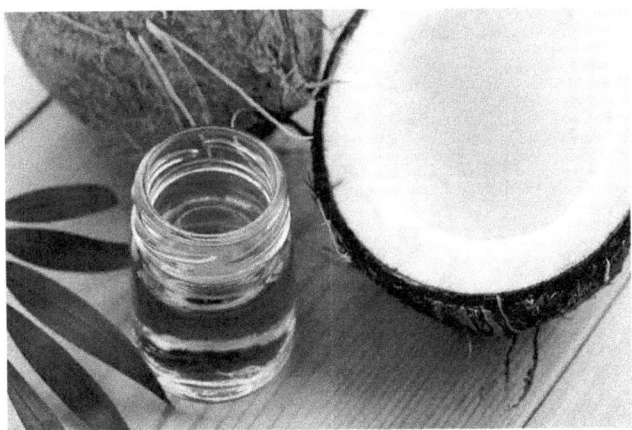

Recipe 02: Roll-on Blend – Mr. Sandman

Ingredients

- 10 ml roller bottle: 1
- Coconut oil: 2 Teaspoons
- Vetiver Essential Oil: 1 Drop
- Royal Sandalwood Essential Oil: 1 Drop
- Waterproof Label: 1

Directions

Add essential oils with coconut oil in the roller bottle. Afterwards, put inside the roller attachment along with its lid. Place the waterproof label and keep away at a safe place.

Recipe 03: Roll-on Blend – Sleepy Head

Ingredients

- 10 ml roller bottle: 1
- Coconut oil: 2 Teaspoons
- Lavender Oil: 1 Drop
- Orange Essential Oil: 1 Drop
- Waterproof Label: 1

Directions

Add essential oils with coconut oil in the roller bottle. Afterwards, put inside the roller attachment along with its lid. Place the waterproof label and keep away at a safe place.

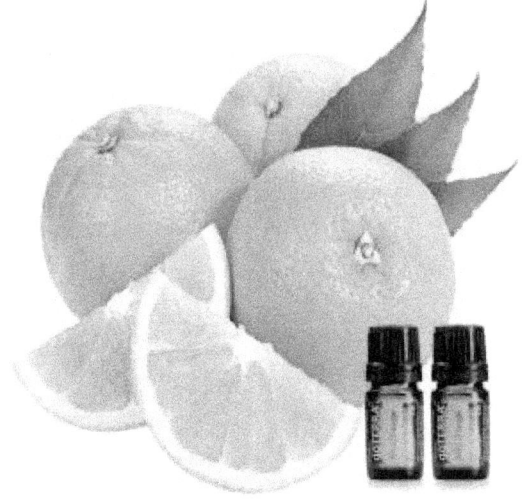

Recipe 04: Immune Booster Blend

Ingredients:

- Melaleuca Essential Oil: 3 Drops
- Oregano Essential Oil: 2 Drops
- Protective Blend: 3 Drops
- Frankincense Essential Oil: 1 Drop
- Carrier Oil: Almond, Jojoba, Etc

Directions:

Before your healthy kids are about to go to bed, a gentle swipe of the blend on the bottom of your child's feet should do the needful. Make sure it's applied regularly before bed for having its effect as an immune booster.

Recipe 05: The Focus Blend For Kids: Great For School-Going Children

Ingredients:

- Peppermint: 3 Drops
- Wild Orange: 3 Drops
- Carrier Oil: Almond, Jojoba, Etc

Directions:

You can apply it on your child's wrist or temples or ask them do it on their own during their school hours. It can be applied on regular intervals throughout the day. It helps staying calm and keep a sharp focus, especially for school-going children.

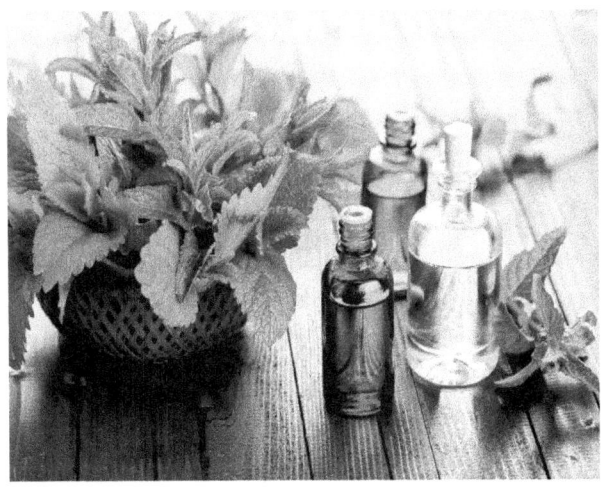

Recipe 06: Roll-On: Anti-Critter

Ingredients:

- Rosemary Essential Oil: 2 Drops
- Melaleuca Essential Oil: 2 Drops
- Eucalyptus Essential Oil: 2 Drops
- Peppermint: 2 Drops
- Carrier Oil: Almond, Jojoba.

Directions:

Roll the mixture on behind the nape of the neck and the ears. It can also be used to roll in your hair and to avoid any bees or wasps from being attracted to the kid's hair. The oil combination has a scent hated by such unwanted guests.

Chapter 2 – DIY Essential Oil Recipes for a Good Night Sleep for All Children

Recipe 07: Good Sleep Boosting Blend:

Ingredients:

- Lemon: 3 Drops
- Oregano: 2 Drops
- Protective Blend: 2 Drops
- Peppermint: 2 Drops
- Clove: 3 Drops
- Melaleuca Essential Oil: 1 Drop
- Carrier Oil: Almond, Jojoba, Etc

Directions:

This powerful essential oil helps your children to get a great sleep at night and wake up as fresh as new the next morning. It would help them get a deep sleep, making them fresh and all set to go the next morning. It can be applied on the child's feet or wrists at night to gain the maximum benefits out of it.

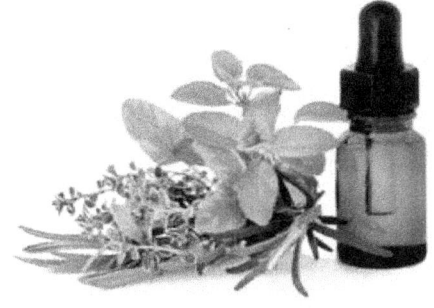

Recipe 8: Super Night Sleep Booster Blend:

Ingredients:

- Melaleuca Essential Oil: 5 Drops
- Oregano: 2 Drops
- Carrier Oil: Almond, Jojoba, Etc
- Protective Blend: 5 Drops
- Frankincense: 2 Drops
- Lemon: 3 Drops

Directions:

This powerful essential oil helps your children to get a great sleep at night and wake up as fresh as new the next morning. It can be applied on the child's feet or wrists at night to gain the maximum benefits out of it. It would help them get a deep sleep, making them fresh and all set to go the next morning.

Recipe 9: Stress Reliever Blend for Kids

Ingredients:

- Peppermint: 8 drops
- Frankincense Essential Oil: 3 drops
- Lavender Essential Oil: 5 drops
- Chamomile Oil: 5 drops
- Carrier Oil: 5 Drops (Almond, Jojoba, Etc)

Directions:

Once the blend is made, it can be applied on the child's nape of neck, forehead and temples. This blend would make sure that your kids get a good deep sleep and wake up relieved with any stress of school or homework.

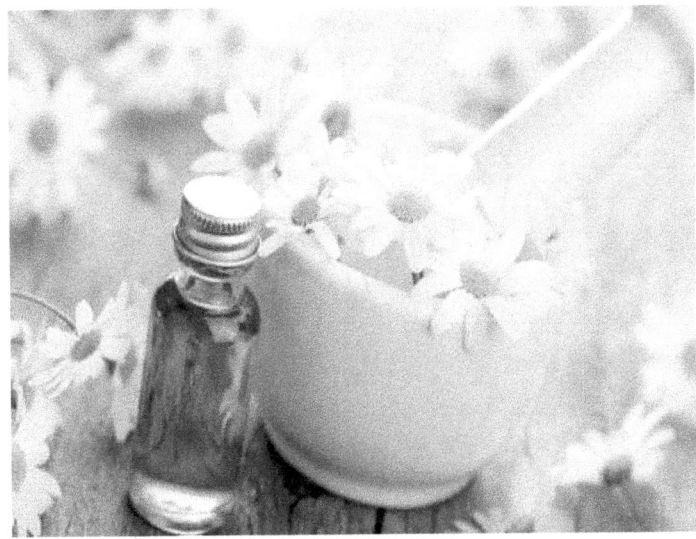

Recipe 10: Sleep Tight – A Good Night Sleep Essential Oil Blend

Ingredients:

- Lavender Essential Oil: 75 Drops
- Sweet Marjoram Essential Oil: 45 Drops
- Roman Chamomile Essential Oil: 30 Drops
- Bergamot Essential Oil: 30 Drops
- Ylang Ylang Essential Oil: 6 Drops
- Valerian Essential Oil: 6 Drops

Directions:

Mix together all the essential oils in a 15 ml bottle and swirl it gently so that all the mixture settles in well with each other. Place a label and keep it in a dark and cool place while not in use with other oils. Your child can use the blend as a smelling salt, aromatherapy inhaler, shower steamers, diffuser in the bedroom or a roll-on. Its proven, your child will have the best sleep ever!

Recipe 11: The Deep Sleep Blend

Ingredients:

- Melaleuca Essential Oil: 1 Drop
- Clove Essential Oil: 3 Drops
- Protective Blend: 2 Drops
- Peppermint Essential Oil: 2 Drops
- Oregano Essential Oil: 2 Drops
- Lemon Essential Oil: 3 Drops
- Carrier Oil: Almond, Jojoba, Etc

Directions:

This blend would make sure that your kids get a good deep sleep and wake up relieved with any stress of school or homework. Mix together all the essential oils in a 15 ml bottle and swirl it gently so that all the mixture settles in well with each other. Once the blend is made, it can be applied on the child's nape of neck, forehead and temples.

Place a label and keep it in a dark and cool place while not in use with other oils. Your child can use the blend as a smelling salt, aromatherapy inhaler, shower steamers, diffuser in the bedroom or a roll-on. It's proven, your child will have the best sleep ever!

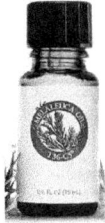

Recipe 12: The Chamomile Sleep Blend:

Ingredients:

- Chamomile Essential Oil: 5 Drops
- Orange Essential Oil: 9 Drops
- Benzoin Essential Oil: 6 Drops
- Moisturizer: 50g

Directions:

Mix these oils well and place them in a bottle. A gentle application on the child's neck and upper chest would help the child sleep deep and is best for kids experiencing nightmares or who frequently get scared.

It's also very effective for kids experiencing insomnia and constipation. It can be used when the kids are bathing and its lovely scent should do the rest while sleeping.

Recipe 13: Cedar wood Calming Recipe

Ingredients:

- Lavender oil – 5 drops
- Cedar wood oil – 5 drops
- Vetiver oil – 5 drops
- Sweet almond oil – 10 drops

Directions:

Get a 5 ml bottle and add the following oils in it such as lavender, cedar wood oil, vetiver oil and sweet almond oil. Blend them together and massage it little on the forehead on your child.

It will keep them calm and they will be able to sleep peacefully with comfort. When they will wake up, they will feel fresh and won't irritate you as much as they used to. Try this and you will be glad that you know this recipe.

Recipe 14: Ylang Ylang Essential Oil Recipe

Ingredients:

- Vetiver – 10 drops
- Lavender – 4 drops
- Ylang Ylang – 4 drops
- Chamomile – 4 drops
- Frankincense oil – 2 drops
- Clary Sage oil – 2 drops
- Marjoram oil – 2 drops
- Coconut oil – 1 tsp.

Directions:

Mix all the ingredients together into a 10 ml bottle. Make sure they all are blend properly and then you can either mix the drop into a diffuser to make it spread all around the house or you can massage your child forehead from it.

This makes an awesome fragrance which you children will surely love so make sure to explain them what it is for and you will see the positive change the next morning.

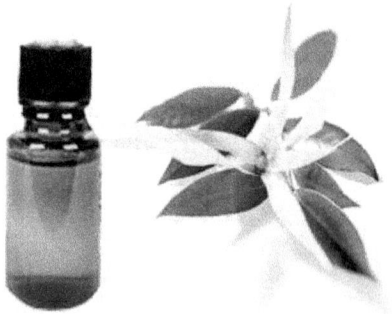

Recipe 15: Mind Calming Blend

Ingredients:

- Frankincense oil – 2 drops
- Pepper mint oil – 3 drops
- Rosemary oil – 4 drops

Directions:

Get a diffuser and add the following ingredients in it such as frankincense oil, pepper mint oil and rosemary oil. Blend it well with the spoon and turn on the diffuser at home.

You will see that you child will be calm and won't be screaming around with disturbing you all the time. it calms their nerves and they are only doing what they want to do without disturbing the mom.

Recipe 16: Lime oil Calming Recipe

Ingredients:

- Peppermint oil – 3 drops
- Lime oil – 4 drops
- Frankincense oil – 4 drops
- Orange essential oil – 6 drops

Directions:

Get a 5 ml bottle and add all the ingredients in it along with water in it. Add peppermint, lime oil, frankincense oil and orange oil together in it. Shake it well and then add the drops into a diffuser. Mix it well.

It will help the child sleep properly without waking up at night again and again. You will see that he/she will be calm than usual.

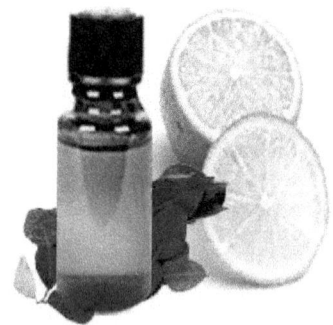

Recipe 17: Grapefruit Calming Recipe

Ingredients:

- Lime oil – 3 drops
- Lemon oil – 5 drops
- Orange oil – 10 drops
- Grapefruit oil – 15 drops
- Lemon grass oil – 10 drops

Directions:

Add all the oils into a 10 ml bottle along with Luke warm bottle. Shake it well and then take the drops in your palm. Blend it in your hand and apply it on your child's forehead. This will help him/her ease up and you will see that their behavior will be changed the next morning when they wake up.

They won't be fussing around much and won't be a pain for you so you can easily use this recipe to keep them calm all day long. Use this regularly and notice the behavior.

Recipe 18: Melissa Oil Recipe

Ingredients:

- Melissa – 10 drops
- Lavender – 10 drops
- Rose – 4 drops

Directions:

Mix all the ingredients in a diffuser and let them spread in the entire house. You do not have to keep your child near it but it will mix into the air which will be inhaled and the child will stay calm. It will keep their head calm and if you wish you can also mix it in a bottle and massage it on their forehead for it to react instantly.

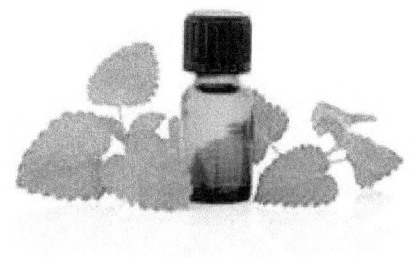

Chapter 4 – Essential Oil Massage Blends for Toddlers

Recipe 19: Sage Oil Massage Recipe for Toddlers

Ingredients:

- Sweet Almond – 10 tbsp.
- Sage – 10 drops
- Marjoram – 5 drops
- Rosemary – 5 drops

Directions:

Get all the ingredients together in the 10 ml bottle and mix them well. After you have mixed them properly then rub it on your hand and massage a little on your toddler body. It will keep the muscles relaxed and they will stay happy most of the times. The essence of essential oils keep their mood light and they do not tend to give you a hard time.

Recipe 20: Bergamot Fun Blend For Massage

Ingredients:

- Lavender oil – 4 drops
- Bergamot oil – 4 drops

Directions:

Mix the ingredients into a 5 ml bottle along with Luke warm water and shake it well. When the mixture is thick and it starts smelling like an essence then lay down your baby and massage the whole body gently.

You will see how happy he/she will get with the massage along with having fun with you.

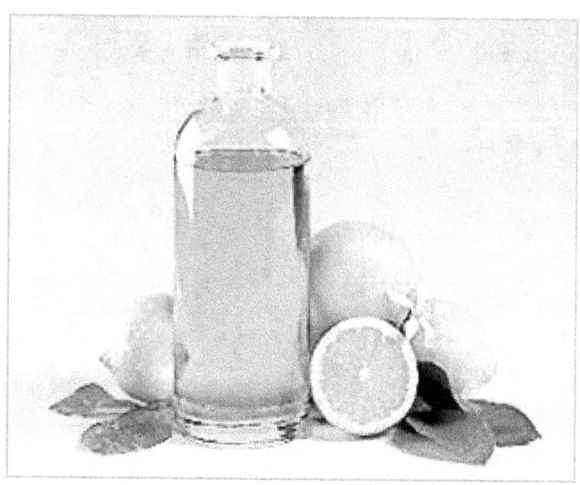

Recipe 21: Juniper Mix Massage Recipe

Ingredients:

- Peppermint – 15 drops
- Black pepper - 15 drops
- Eucalyptus - 15 drops
- Ginger - 15 drops
- Juniper Berry - 15 drops

Directions:

Blend all the ingredients into a bottle and shake it well. Keep it aside for a while and then massage your toddler's forehead with it gently. Make sure that you do it carefully and it does not touch their eyes.

It will have a calming and soothing effect on the baby's body with making them fresh. They won't get lazy and stay active all the time with being engaged with themselves.

Recipe 22: Sweet Almond Mix

Ingredients:

- Sweet Almond
- Rosemary (3 drops)
- Sweet marjoram (4 drops)
- Ginger (1 drop)
- Roman chamomile (6 drops)

Directions:

This is a complete warm body massage for the toddler. Make sure you keep them covered after its application. Mix the ingredients together into a 5 ml bottle along with Luke warm water. Shake it well and then get few drops on your palm.

Massage the whole body of your toddler gently and keep them warm after that for about an hour. It will make them feel easy and relaxed without getting tired and they will not irritate you as well.

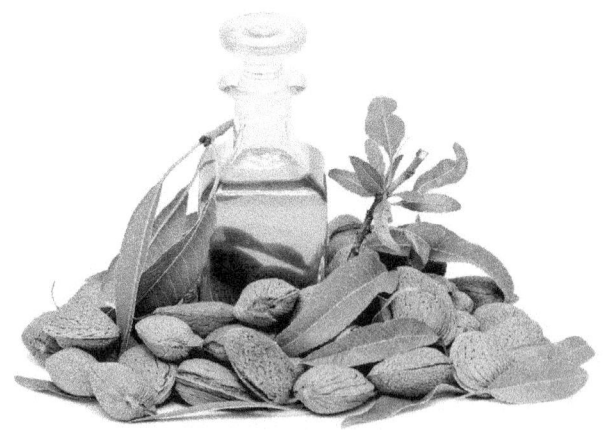

Recipe 23: Coconut oil Massage Therapy

Ingredients:

- Coconut oil (2 tbsp.)
- Sweet marjoram (2 drops)
- Cinnamon (10 drops)
- Peppermint (5 drops)
- Lavender (15 drops)

Directions:

Get a 10 ml bottle and add Luke warm water in it. Mix all the essential oils in it and shake it well. Keep it aside for a while for it settle.

Take some drop and cover your hands with it by applying it on the whole body of your toddler. He/she will feel better and you will see that they won't be crying much as well. They will feel relaxed as long as you are giving them food and staying around them. You can do work in your kitchen and they will be playing on their own without any disturbance.

Recipe 24: Eucalyptus Essential Oil Massage

Ingredients:

- Eucalyptus – 5 drops
- Lavender – 15 drops
- Ginger – 10 drops

Directions:

Get a 5 ml bottle and these essential oils drops in it. Shake it well and then add Luke warm water in it. Keep it aside for about an hour and then massage the forehead of your baby with this. You can massage the feet bottom with it as well to give the relaxing feel to the baby to take away their tiredness. You will see that they will fall asleep within some time because they will feel relaxed and easy on their head.

Sometimes the babies irritate because they want parents to be with them all the time but this massage will help them stay normal even if you are doing your house chores and he/she is playing on his own.

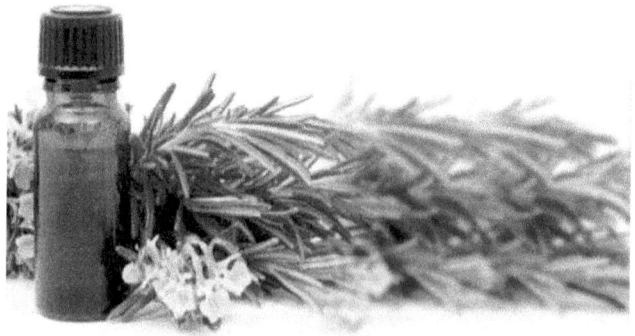

Chapter 5 – Essential Oil Blends to Protect Children from Allergies and Infections

Recipe 25: Clove Recipe Blend for Allergy

Ingredients:

- Clove – 2 drops
- Lavender – 3 drops
- Peppermint – 3 drops
- Birch – 2 drops
- Thyme – 2 drops

Directions:

Mix all the ingredients in a bowl and add them into a diffuser. Turn on the diffuser at night time or when you wake up in the morning which will be inhaled by the children. It will help them decrease the allergies and they won't be having any headaches or pains.

Recipe 26: Ginger Magic Blend

Ingredients:

- Marjoram – 15 drops
- Lavender – 15 drops
- Ginger – 10 drops
- Rosemary – 15 drops

Directions:

Add all the ingredients in a 5 ml bottle and shake it well. Keep it aside to settle and then add it into a diffuser for the essence to spread all around the house. This will help your child stay away from the bacteria and infections which they can catch.

The essence is inhaled and causes the body to heal and remove any bacteria from the body by flushing it out and giving a rest to the brain as well.

Recipe 27: Yarrow Oil Blend

Ingredients:

- Yarrow – 3 drops
- Clove oil – 10 drops
- Peppermint – 10 drops

Directions:

The yarrow oil helps to relieve allergies quickly so add it with clove oil and peppermint oil in a 5 ml bottle and shake it well. Turn on the diffuser and add the drops into it to have the essence spread in the house.

When the essence is inhaled, it helps to keep the children calm from fussing if they are not feeling well and also heals then inside with the treatment of natural ingredients.

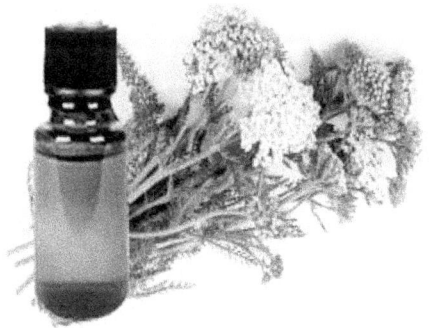

Recipe 28: Black Pepper Blend

Ingredients:

- Ginger – 20 drops
- Cinnamon – 12 drops
- Black pepper – 12 drops

Directions:

Black pepper is the best for the allergies to calm so add them with ginger and cinnamon in a 10 ml bottle by shaking it well. You can use it both ways by massing it over the forehead of your child gently or by adding the drops into the diffuser.

Recipe 29: Cypress Remedy Blend

Ingredients:

- Sweet Almond – 14 tbsp.
- Sweet marjoram – 20 drops
- Cypress – 12 drops
- Ginger – 4 drops

Directions:

Add all the ingredients in a 10 ml bottle with Luke warm water in it. Mix them well by shaking the bottle thoroughly. When done, add the drops into the diffuser to help you child get some relieve from the allergies.

The healing power of the essential oils helps the nerves to calm down and fixes any infection which is minor without any further step.

Recipe 30: Sweet Marjoram Recipe

Ingredients:

- Roman chamomile – 10 drops
- Sweet marjoram – 5 drops
- Lavender oil – 3 drops

Directions:

Mix all the ingredients in a bottle and shake them well. Make sure that you keep it aside for a while for the oils to blend in each other. It works as the best treatment for the child who is sneezing all day long. Gives a warm feel when inhaled through the diffuser.

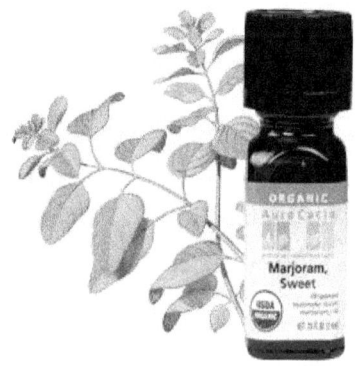

Conclusion

If you are someone who is new to the world of essential oils, then it is better to start with the lighter ones. The fragrance may seem too strong in the beginning if you jump to the clove scent because it is strong and may be a reason for your headache at one point. A list of all the possible blends is available for you in the eBook which is easy to make. You simply need to have the water and add the oils in it. There is no proper direction for each but the similar procedure for you to follow.

The essential oils fragrance works like magic for those who stay stress from their busy lives and makes your pains go away. Life becomes tough, and we tend to forget how actually to manage it so then comes the main role of the essential oils which soothes your brain and gives you some peace to your kids. You can relax and massage on your child's body easily at any time with the essential oils blends.

It depends on the size of the jar in which you are making the blends but mostly people try the small ones, and the instructions are based on that also. You can try any of these recipes at your home, and you will see how peaceful it will be. They work wonders and keeps your child calm in your daily life routine without any disturbance. Once you start liking the essence of it, you will be glad that you have this eBook to try other new blends. This eBook is full of awesome recipes to try on your kids which are safe and will always have a positive effect on your kids.

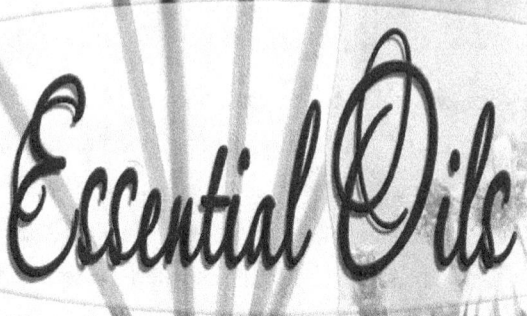

Essential Oils

35

Essential Oils Blends
Every Beginner Should Try

Lora Brenner

Essential Oils:

35 Essential Oils Blends Every Beginner

Should Try

Introduction

Essential oils can be used for physical and emotional wellness. You can use single essential oil or use complex blends by your experience and desired results. You should select quality essential oils to get the advantage of their original properties.

Almost all essential oils are safe for external use, but a couple of brands are ideal for internal use. Some therapeutic grade brands are suitable for medicinal use.

Some brands of essential oils have additives or fillers. Try to use pure essential oils to get desired benefits. Some pure essential oils are clary sage, rosemary, lemongrass, bergamot, eucalyptus, tea tree, pine, cypress, basil, and lemon, grapefruit and ginger essential oils.

The chemical and physical properties of elastic aromatic properties of essential oil enable them to smoothly move through air and interact with olfactory sensors in your nose. These unique features make all essential oils ideal for aromatherapy and massage on your body parts.

Blending can be difficult for beginners, but there is no need to worry because the essential oils are grouped together by their fragrance. You can blend oils of similar categories and match them. Essential oils are divided into following categories:

- Woodsy: Cedar and Pine

- Flora: Jasmine, Neroli and Lavender

- Herbaceous: Basil, Rosemary and Marjoram

- Earthy: Patchouli, Vetiver and Oakmoss

- Medicinal: Tea Tree, Cajuput and Eucalyptus

- Minty: Spearmint and Peppermint

- Oriental: Patachouli and Ginger

- Spicy: Cinnamon, Clove and Nutmeg

- Citrus: Lime, Lemon and Orange

Famous Blending Categories

- Floral are good to blend with citrus, spicy and woodsy

- Earthy blends well with minty and woodsy

- Woodsy are good to blend with citrus, oriental, spicy, medicinal, minty, herbaceous, earthy and floral

- Minty blends are good for citrus, herbaceous, earthy and woodsy

- Herbaceous blends are excellent for minty and woodsy

- Medicinal blends well with woodsy

- Oriental blends well with citrus, spicy, woodsy and floral

- Spicy oils are good to blend with citrus, oriental, woodsy and floral

- Citrus oils blend well with oriental, spicy, minty, woodsy and floral

Essential oil "note" is based on its evaporation level because after some hours, some essential oils may evaporate and the smell of blend will change.

Top Notes

- Bergamot

- Basil

- Grapefruit

- Eucalyptus

- Lemon

- Peppermint

- Lemongrass

- Spearmint

Middle Notes

- Cypress

- Pine

- Clary sage

- Rosemary

- Tea tree

Base Notes

- Ginger

In this book, you will find 35 essential oil recipes that prove good for you to improve your overall health.

Chapter 1 – Essential Oils to Improve Your Mood

The essential oils are really powerful, and you can use them to treat anxiety. The smell of essential oils quite relaxing and it will help you to soothe your nerves. Smell receptors of your nose can communicate with the parts of your brain to treat your anxiety. The amygdala and hippocampus are the storehouses of your brain for your emotions and memories.

The molecules of essential oils can stimulate these particular parts of your brain and improve your physical and mental health. If you are dealing with anxious feelings, then it is important to use essential oils because these are better to use as compared to medicines. Following are some essential oils that you can use to treat your anxiety:

Tips to Diffuse Your Blend

You can increase the amount of blend by adding your oil in a dark colored bottle made of glass and then roll the bottle between your hands. You can add a diffuser like olive oil to diffuse the blend and use this blend in your bath water.

Carrier Oils

The carrier oils are often used as a diffuser to diffuse the intensity of carrier oils. You can mix these oils with essential oils to take aromatherapy. Following are some famous and frequently used carrier oils:

- Sweet almond oil
- Olive oil
- Sunflower oil

In short, the seed, vegetable, and nut oils can be used to dilute the concentrated essential oils.

Balance Essential Oil

This essential oil is a blend of rosewood, blue tansy, spruce, and frankincense. It is an ideal essential oil to treat your anxiety. You can get a feeling of calmness with the use of this oil. It is a natural remedy used to calm down your nerves and promote the relaxation. The chamomile is used to soothe your nerves. The Frankincense can promote your relaxation and relieve the feelings of sorrow.

Lavender Essential Oil

If you are dealing with anxiousness, then you can try the lavender essential oil. Its scent is really calm and attractive, and you can use it in the water while taking a bath. You can also add it few drops in the deodorant to make it relaxing. There are a number of scientific proves that the lavender can reduce the anxiety and enhance the mood of patients.

Wild Orange Essential Oils

Wild orange essential oil is a great choice to reduce anxiety and boost your mood. It can increase your happiness and well-being. It is not good to eat any essential oil, but you can add a few drops of orange essential oils in your recipe to enhance citrus flavor.

Serenity Essential Oil

Serenity is a useful essential oil prepared to treat your anxiety. You can combine this essential oil with the lavender, sweet marjoram, ylang-ylang, sandalwood, and vanilla. These all oils have excellent properties, and you can take massage of these oils to promote sleep. The ylang-ylang is really beneficial for your central nervous system. The serenity can be applied topically or you may diffuse it in the air. You can apply it to the bottom of your feet before going to bed to enjoy a deep and relaxing sleep.

Bergamot Essential Oil

The bergamot is used to relieve the tension and stress, and it can also be used to improve the health of your skin. It features citrus scent and you can use it to enhance your mood. The bergamot can promote the relaxation by reducing the feelings of anxiousness. It is the best essential oil to apply to the skin or diffuse in the air to treating the tension and promote a good sleep. In order to enhance the benefits of essential oils, it will be good to use magnesium supplement to overcome your anxious feelings.

Grounding Blend

It is a useful blend of howood, spruce, frankincense and chamomile. If you are suffering from anxiety and tension, then this blend will really help you. It can promote the feelings of calmness and reduce your stress.

Application

The grounding blend can be applied to your feet on a regular basis. You can also massage it over the back of your neck, heart and the wrists get better results.

Apply on the wrists and rub them together and inhale. You can mix this oil with a calming blend to increase its benefits.

Respiratory Blend

It is a versatile blend used for all respiratory issues. It is a combination of peppermint, lemon, ravensara lead, melaleuca and Cardamom seeds. It will help you to calm down your brain during anxiety.

Application:

Apply a few drops on your chest to relax your nerves and open your airways for relaxed breathing.

Frankincense

It is a king of essential oils that is why it is really valuable to slow down the fear, anxiety and tension. If you are suffering from stressful feelings, then it is an excellent choice for you. It can help you to combat the feelings of fear and anxiety.

Directions:

It is great oil for regular use because it can promote your cellular balance. It can reduce feelings of anxiety, so use it in the diffuse state. You can inhale it, or massage your feet and back with a few drops of oil. Its blend with lavender oil and wild orange can help you to get rid of anxiety.

Try a Joyful Blend

The smell of this oil will be great to treat the feelings of anxiety and tensions. It can treat anxiety and depression at the same time. The blend contains lavender, tangerine, elemi, lemon, Melissa, ylang-ylang, sandalwood, and osmanthus.

Directions:

You can apply it on your heart, bones, behind the ear, neck, forehead and wrists to reduce stress. Its regular application will help you to calm your mind and get rid of tensions.

Lemon Essential Oil

It is versatile oil with lots of benefits because of its properties. The lemon oil is excellent to uplift your mood, revive your stressful feelings, and stimulate your feelings.

The lemon enhances the sense of security and trust. It can help you to remove confusions and tensions. It can clear the obstacles and improve your feelings.

Directions:

You can use it on a regular basis in water. Just add 1 drop of essential oil in a glass of water and then use it for the whole day.

Calming Blend

If you want to promote relaxed feelings, then this blend is excellent for you. It can control your anger and promote good health with calmness. The blend contains sweet marjoram, lavender, ylang-ylang, roman chamomile, sandalwood, and vanilla bean.

Direction:

Use almost 5 drops of this blend in the hot water for relaxation. You can also apply it on the back of your neck and inhale it through a diffuser. Some drops should be applied to the bottoms of your feet before going to sleep. It's awesome smell can leave excellent effects on your nerves.

Patchouli Essential Oil

It is a special oil to harmonize your mind and keep it stable without any tension. It can reduce the negative thoughts by relieving the depression and increase the joy in your life. You can recover from tension, stress and tiredness of mind.

Direction:

You can apply a diffused form of this oil to the base of your skull. Inhale the aroma of the oil to calm your fortitude and reduce disorganized thoughts.

Chapter 2 – Coconut EO Blends for Hair Problems

Coconut oil is equipped with antioxidants and antibacterial properties. You can improve the health of your scalp and promote the growth of healthy hair. It has the ability to fight with infections and add volume and extra shine to your hair. There are some amazing uses of coconut oil:

Natural Conditioner

Coconut oil is a natural conditioner that helps you to avoid damage while combing your hair. It is safe for delicate and sensitive skins of children. You can condition your hair with coconut oil easily:

Take a ¼ teaspoon of liquid coconut oil to start oiling your short hair. If your hair are thick and long, you can start with a ½ tablespoon of oil on your palm. Try to use sparingly on thin hair to make them healthy.

After washing your hair with a gentle shampoo, you can apply a small amount of oil on your hair. 1 teaspoon is enough for short hair and 2 teaspoons coconut oil is enough on medium hair. If your hair are extra-long, you can take 1 tablespoon or more after rubbing in your palms. Now cover your hair with a shower cap for 1 to 2 hours or for the whole night. Use a natural shampoo to wash your hair. If you want to treat your damaged and dry hair, you can add a few drops of sandalwood oil (Essential oil).

Trigger Hair Growth

Coconut oil can improve the blood circulation and you can get positive results with a gentle massage of 10 minutes almost three times a week. One teaspoon oil is enough for your scalp only.

To deep condition your hair, you can add a few drops of chamomile oil, sandalwood oil, and coconut oil. This mixture will increase the blood circulation in the scalp for amazing results. After a massage on your scalp, you can cover your hair with the shower cap to let the scalp absorb oils. It is good for all types of hair and improve the health of the follicles.

Get Rid of Dandruff

Coconut oil is good to fight with dandruff by killing the virus, bacteria and other harmful elements on the scalp. You can use one of these oils, such as tea tree oil, Cedarwood oil, lavender oil, rosemary oil and wintergreen oil.

Take one of these oils and prepare a mixture of 5 drops of essential oil and 2 drops of coconut oil to massage your scalp. Use a shower cap to cover your head for 30 minutes and wash with a gentle shampoo. You can repeat this procedure three times in a week.

Coconut Oil Treatment for Lice

The coconut oil is good for the prevention of lices and you can prepare a mixture of coconut oil with other ingredients. You can make a blend of coconut oil (3 tablespoons) and tea tree and ylang-ylang oils (1 teaspoon each). You can increase the amount of oil for long hair.

Rub this mixture into your scalp and comb your hair with a smooth comb. Use a shower cap to cover your head and wait for two hours. You can sit in the sun or use keep your shower cap warm with the periodic use of hair dryer. After this, carefully remove your shower cap and keep in a sealed bag. After this, comb your hair and rinse your hair carefully.

After washing hair, you can prepare a mixture of 1 cup water and 2 cups vinegar (apple cider vinegar). Spray half bottle on your hair and scalp, but keep your eyes always close. The remaining mixture should be drizzled on the hair after leaning on the sink.

Once again, wash your hair and comb them with a smooth comb. After this, apply coconut oil on your scalp and cover your hair with a shower cap. If you want, you can style it as per your needs and leave the oil in the hair until your next wash. To increase the effectiveness of this treatment, you should repeat it once between 5 and 10 days for a few weeks.

Chapter 3 – EO Blends for Weight Loss

You can use coconut essential oil and grapefruit essential oil, you can use essential oils to reduce weight.

Include Liquid Coconut Oil in Your Diet

- If your weight is between 90 and 130 pounds, you can use almost 1 tablespoon of oil 3 times a day.

- If your weight is between 131 and 180 pounds, you can include 1.5 tablespoons of oil 3 times a day before taking meals.

- If your weight is more than 180 pounds, you can include 2 tablespoons of oil in your diet and take it thrice a day. You can drink 2 tablespoons oil before every meal.

Herbal Tea with Coconut Oil

You can use liquid coconut oil on a regular basis, such as mix one or two tablespoons of oil in a cup of hot water. One gram of coconut contains 9 calories; therefore, you can control your calories while including it in your diet. Two tablespoons of coconut oils are enough in a cup of green tea. Mix it well and enjoy on a regular basis to get rid of obesity.

Coconut Oil and Lemon

The combination of lemon and coconut oil can be a great solution to melt your body fat. Take the juice of one whole lemon in a glass of hot water and mix it well. You can take this water on a regular basis in the morning. This will help you blast your body fat.

Boost Your Metabolism with Coconut Diet

Almost one ounce of coconut oil can help your body to burn 120 calories extra on a regular basis. The coconut oil can help you to boost your metabolism level; therefore, you should consume almost 3 ounces coconut oil on a regular basis. It will be better to select virgin coconut oil because it is extracted from fresh coconut meat and milk.

Include Coconut Oil in Regular Diet

If you are fond of cakes, muffins, brownies and cookies, you can make them healthier with coconut oil. The vegetables can be cooked in a mixture of coconut oil and lemon juice. You can enhance the taste of popcorn with the help of coconut oil instead of butter. It can be an important part of your smoothies and morning coffee to trigger your weight loss speed.

Morning and Evening Smoothies with Grapefruit Oil

If you want to enjoy fresh smoothies, take 18 ounces coconut milk and mix with 1 teaspoon of grapefruit oil and 10 ounces of water. You can blend these ingredients in a mixer and to enhance its flavor, add a cup of strawberries.

Blend these ingredients well and add natural sweetener as per your taste. You can enjoy it regularly with some additions, such as change strawberries with blueberries.

Mixture of Water, Coconut Oil, and Pineapple

You can try this smoothie regularly to reduce weight and it is really healthy for your body. It is really simple to make:

A cup of coconut water and 2 tablespoons of virgin oil is good to make a mixture. You can enhance its flavor by adding ½ cup blueberries, ½ cup of pineapples and a handful of spinach. Make sure to add a few cubes of ice and blend all ingredients. Blend these ingredients in a mixer and add a natural sweetener to enhance its taste. It can increase your energy and help you to reduce weight

Chapter 4 – Reduce Depression and Stress with EO Blends

If you want a peaceful and calm atmosphere, there are a few sprays that will be useful for you. These blends are good for your health:

Soothing Blends:

Following are some blends that will help you to promote the feelings of relaxation and enhance your mood:

Blend 01:

- 1 drop Rose
- 3 drops Orange
- 1 drop Vetiver

Mix all these essential oils and pour it in the water before taking a bath. It will help you to reduce anger.

Blend 02:

- 3 drops Bergamot
- 1 drop Ylang Ylang
- 1 drop Jasmine

Add this blend in your bath water and take a bath with it to gradually reduce your anger.

Blend 03:

- 1 drop Roman Chamomile
- 2 drops Bergamot
- 2 Drops Orange Essential Oil

Take a relaxing bath after adding this blend in a bucket of water, and get the benefits of this bath.

Blend 04:

- 3 drops of Orange Essential Oil
- 2 drops of Patchouli Oil

This will be the relaxing blend for to manage your anger. Include it in a bucket of water to take a bath.

Tips to Diffuse Your Blend

You can increase the amount of blend by adding your oil in a dark colored bottle made of glass and then roll the bottle between your hands. You can add a diffuser like olive oil to diffuse the blend and use this blend in your bath water.

Carrier Oils

The carrier oils are often used as a diffuser to diffuse the intensity of carrier oils. You can mix these oils with essential oils to take aromatherapy. Following are some famous and frequently used carrier oils:

- Sweet almond oil
- Olive oil
- Sunflower oil

In short, the seed, vegetable, and nut oils can be used to dilute the concentrated essential oils.

Rose Essential Oils

The rose essential oils are famous for its properties because it can be used as an antidepressant, antiseptic, antispasmodic, hepatic, uterine, stomachic, etc. The rose essential oil works well to alleviate stress, mental tension, depression, nervous ailments and various other problems. If you want to get rid of anger and mental stress, then use rose essential oil to manage this situation.

Directions:

Take a few drops of diffused rose essential oil and add them in the water. Take a bath with this water on a regular basis. You will notice a gradual change in your anger.

Palo Santo Essential Oil

The palo santo essential oil is used to manage anger because its scent can keep your mind free from worries and tensions. Its anti-inflammatory properties can help you to avoid cancer as well. The regular use of this oil will help you to manage anger and stress.

Directions:

- 5 drops Cedarwood Atlas
- 4 drops Palo Santo
- 1 drop Patchouli
- 5 drops of Bergamot

Make a blend of these essential oils and apply it on the palms of your hands before going to head. Rub your hands and take a deep breath. You can massage your lower back and sole of the feet with the tips of your finger. You will notice a great difference in your condition after taking a massage with this blend.

Mood Enhancing Spray

- Lime: 90 drops
- Eucalyptus: 10 drops
- Emulsifier: 5 ml
- Peppermint: 50 drops
- Distilled water: 4 oz

Make a blend of all essential oils, distilled water and emulsifier, and pour it into a bottle. Make sure to shake well before spraying it in your room. You can use these blends in a diffuser as well by omitting the water and emulsifier. Just make a blend of oils and add a few drops in your diffuser.

Room Fragrance

- Petitgrain: 15 drops
- Lime: 60 drops
- Bergamot: 60 drops
- Emulsifier: 1 teaspoon
- Patchouli: 10 drops
- Tangerine: 30 drops
- Distilled water: 4 ounces

Make a blend of all essential oils, distilled water and emulsifier, and pour it into a bottle. Make sure to shake well before spraying it in your room. This blend can be cloudy, but don't worry because it is normal.

Odor Removal Spray

- Petitgrain: 40 drops

- Pure Water: 4 oz

- Peppermint: 40 drops

- Grapefruit: 40 drops

- Lime: 30 drops

Make a blend of all essential oils, distilled water and emulsifier, and pour it into a bottle. Make sure to shake well before spraying it in your room. Spray in your air for an amazing aroma.

Amazing Carpet Freshener

- Eucalyptus: 30 drops

- Cinnamon Leaf: 30 drops

- Lemongrass: 30 drops

- Clove bud: 10 drops

- Bicarbonate soda aka baking soda: 1/2 cup

Use a wide mouth jar with a lid to add all essential oils and soda. Shake it and let it sit for almost 24 hours. Sprinkle it on the carpet and wait for 15 minutes before vacuuming.

Bathroom Air Fresher

- Peppermint: 25 drops

- Lavender: 5 drops

- Sandalwood: 10 drops

- Distilled Water: One Ounce

You can add these essential oils in plastic bottles used for spray and add water. Now, shake well and spray in your bathroom.

Mood Enhancer Spray

- 3 drops clary sage oil

- 1 drop lemon oil

- 1 drop lavender oil

Make a blend of these oils and add in your diffuser to improve the air quality of your room.

Kill Odor

- 2 drops roman chamomile oil
- 2 drops lavender oil
- 1 drop vetiver oil

Make a blend of these oils and add in your diffuser to improve the air quality of your room.

Relieve Stress

- 3 drops bergamot oil
- 1 drop geranium oil
- 1 drop frankincense oil

Make a blend of these oils and add in your diffuser to improve the air quality of your room.

Reduce Tension and Anxiety

- 3 drops grapefruit oil

- 1 drop jasmine oil

- 1 drop ylang-ylang oil

Make a blend of these oils and add in your diffuser to improve the air quality of your room.

Natural Spring Scent

- Distilled water: 1.5 ounces

- Vodka: 1.5 ounces

- Your Favorite Essential Oil: 20 to 40 drops

- Spray bottle of 4 ounces

Prepare a mixture of all these ingredients and shake vigorously. Spray it in your home for fresh air.

Floral Room Spray

- Ylang Ylang: 10 drops

- Rose Oil: 6 drops

- Sweet orange: 10 drops

- Cardamom: 4 drops

- Distilled Water: One Ounce

Make a blend of these oils and add in your spray bottle. You can also add a few drops of oils in a diffuser to improve the air quality of your room.

Green Earth Spray

- Juniper: 8 drops

- Rosemary: 6 drops

- Jasmine: 6 drops

- Frankincense: 4 drops

You can also add a few drops of oils in a diffuser to improve the air quality of your room. To make its spray, you can add distilled water and alcohol in essential oils.

Energy Boosting Spray

- Lemon oil: 20 drops

- Eucalyptus: 8 drops

- Cinnamon: 2 drops

- Peppermint: 2 drops

You can also add a few drops of oils in a diffuser to improve the air quality of your room. To make its spray, you can add distilled water and alcohol in essential oils.

Citrus Room Spray for Winter

- Cinnamon: 12 drops

- Sweet orange: 12 drops

- Clove: 6 drops

You can also add a few drops of oils in a diffuser to improve the air quality of your room. To make its spray, you can add distilled water and alcohol in essential oils.

Motivating Spray

- Lime: 12 drops

- Ylang ylang: 12 drops

- Rose: 6 drops

You can also add a few drops of oils in a diffuser to improve the air quality of your room. To make its spray, you can add distilled water and alcohol in essential oils.

Note: To make sprays, you should add 1.5 ounces pure distilled water and 1.5 oz witch hazel or vodka. It will help you to improve the strength of your scent.

Chapter 5 – EO Recipes to Use as Room Fresheners

There are some blends that you can use as room freshener to get the advantage of

Air Freshener Spray

- Sage: 25 drops

- Marjoram: 25 drops

- Clove bud: 25 drops

- Spearmint: 25 drops

- Patchouli: 20 drops

- Distilled water: 4 ounces

Prepare a mixture of distilled water and oil, shake well and pour into a spray bottle. You should shake well before use.

Light Air Freshener

- Lavender: 15 drops

- Orange: 10 drops

- Lemon: 10 drops

- Grapefruit: 10 drops

- Lime: 6 drops

- Nutmeg: 3 drops

- Distilled water: 2 ounces

- 4 to 5 ml Emulsifier

Blend oils, distilled water and emulsifier in a spray bottle and shake well to mix this blend. This will be an excellent air freshener to remove pet odor.

Spice Air Freshener

- Sage: 25 drops

- Marjoram: 25 drops

- Clove: 25 drops

- Spearmint: 25 drops

- Emulsifier: 5 ml

- Patchouli: 25 drops

- Distilled water: 4 oz

Make a blend of oils, distilled water, emulsifier and all other ingredients. Pour into spray bottle and shake well before use.

Carpet Spray

- Eucalyptus: 30 drops
- Cinnamon Leaf: 30 drops
- Clove Bud: 10 drops
- Lemongrass: 30 drops
- bicarbonate soda (also known as baking soda): 1/2 cup

Blend all ingredients in a wide bottle and pour it into a spray bottle. Leave it for almost 24 hours. Shake well before use and spray on your carpet almost 15 minutes before vacuum.

Carpet Spray 02

- Juniper Berry: 25 drops
- Cedarwood: 25 drops
- Pure distilled water: 4 ounces
- Pine: 75 drops

Make a blend and shake well this mixture. Pour in the spray bottles and mist in the air.

Christmas Spray

- Orange: 20 drops

- Cinnamon: 30 drops

- Clove Bud: 40 drops

- Ginger: 30 drops

- Distilled water: 4 ounces

Make a blend and shake this mixture well. You can pour this blend into a spray bottle. This spray can improve the atmosphere of your house.

Blend to Improve Air Quality

- Grapefruit: 6 drops

- Spearmint: 4 drops

Make a blend and shake this mixture well. You can pour this blend into a spray bottle. This spray can improve the atmosphere of your house. This blend can be added in a diffuser.

Calming Spray

- Cajuput: 30 drops

- Marjoram: 30 drops

- Lavender: 30 drops

- Vetiver: 30 drops

- Petitgrain: 30 drops

- Pure water: 4 ounces

Make a blend and shake this mixture well. You can pour this blend into a spray bottle and in a diffuser. This spray can be helpful to calm overactive kids. This can be sprayed in the evening before they sleep.

Spray for Pet Odors

- Lavender: 10 drops

- Orange: 10 drops

- Geranium: 5 drops

- Lemon: 5 drops

- Nutmeg: 2 drops

- Tea tree: 6 drops

- Neroli: 3 drops

Prepare a blend of all these ingredients and add 4 to 5 drops in a diffuser.

Pillow Spray for Sweet Dreams

- Distilled water: 15 ml

- Lavender: 2 drops

- Chamomile: 1 drop

- Orange: 1 drop

- Ylang ylang: 1 drop

Make a blend of all ingredients and shake them well. Spray on your pillow cases and enjoy a comfortable sleep.

Alertness Spray

- Bergamot: 40 drops

- Grapefruit: 40 drops

- Peppermint: 40 drops

- Juniper Berry: 30 drops

- Lavender: 25 drops

- Pure water: 4 ounces

Mix all ingredients, shake well and pour into any mist sprayer.

Alertness Spray for Spray Bottle

- Bergamot: 2 drops

- Distilled water: 2 ounces

- Frankincense: 2 drops

- Lemon: 2 drops

- Citronella: 2 drops

- Lavender: 4 drops

Pour all these ingredients in a bottle, shake this blend well and spray in your house. You shouldn't spray it on the furniture.

Freshener Spray

- Clove: 30 drops

- Bergamot: 10 drops

- Nutmeg: 5 drops

- Orange: 40 drops

- Cinnamon: 5 drops

- Ginger: 5 drops

- Lemon: 5 drops

Blend all oils and pour 12 drops of this blend into one ounce lukewarm distilled water, shake it well and spray it in your room.

Spicy Air Freshener

- Sage: 25 drops

- Marjoram: 25 drops

- Spearmint: 25 drops

- Patchouli: 25 drops

- Clove: 25 drops

- Distilled water: 4 oz

- Emulsifier: 5 ml

Make a blend of all oils and emulsifier, and add distilled water in this blend. Shake it well and let it sit for one day. Now, spray it in your rooms.

Air Freshener 02

- Grapefruit: 50 drops

- Distilled water: 4 oz

- Orange: 10 drops

- Lime: 50 drops

- Emulsifier: 5 ml

- Patchouli: 10 drops

Make a blend of all essential oils, distilled water and emulsifier, and pour it into a bottle. Make sure to shake well before spraying it in your room. You can use these blends in a diffuser as well by omitting the water and emulsifier. Just make a blend of oils and add a few drops in your diffuser.

Conclusion

Lots of essential oils may help you to deal with these emotions. You can control your anger by taking a bath, vaporizations and a massage with a few drops of essential oils. The great essential oils are orange essential oil, ginger essential oil, rose essential oil, tea tree essential oil, rose essential oils, chamomile essential oil and lots of others.

The regular use of these oils will help you to surpass anger, get rid of anxiety, reduce sorrows, increase happiness and make your life easy. You should read the precautions before using any essential oil. Consult your doctor and do a patch test to know if it is the right choice for you.

It is important to be very careful while ingesting essential oils and consult your doctor. In the case of any irritation or nausea feelings, stop the use of essential oils and increase the water intake. The excessive water will remove the toxic substances of the oil from your body.

Herbal Antibiotics

35 DIY Natural Holistic Herbal Remedies
For Preventing and Healing Illnesses

by Maria George

Herbal Antibiotics:

35 Natural Holistic Herbal Remedies For

Preventing And Healing Illnesses

Introduction

There you are, browsing the aisles in another department store, trying to find the one antibiotic that's going to work for you. Of course, if you want to use something prescription strength, you have to go to the doctor, but that costs money.

Then you have to wait in line to fill your prescription, and you have to pay a lot more money for the prescription itself. No matter how you look at it, you are pouring hundreds of dollars into a single doctor's visit, without a lot to show for it.

This is going to lead to more and more issues, as you have to deal with medical bills, time off from work, and the synthetic material you are putting into your body. That's right, even the medication that is supposed to be helping you could be doing more harm than good if it's not used properly.

Your body is designed to use the natural, and when you aren't putting that into your body, then you are subjecting your body to things you don't want it to be subjected to. You know how a single substance can affect every part of your life, and it doesn't seem to matter what your initial ailment was, you can end up with several other issues as a result of using the antibiotics.

But, if you go all natural, you don't have to worry about these things. Forget side effects, forget the other issues that can creep into your life if you aren't careful, and forget basing your treatment on other things you are doing. If you have an infection, you want to take care of something, or you simply want to keep all natural medication on hand, growing your own herbal supplements is the answer.

However, if you have never done this before, you could be facing a lot more questions. What kinds of supplements do you need? Where are you going to get these herbs? How do you store them... or grow them in the first place? How do you use them?

And others. But, with this book, you are going to learn the answers to these questions, and more. I am going to show you how to use the natural world around you to your greatest benefit, and show you just what you need to do to say goodbye to synthetic medication for good.

This book is going to change your life, and you are going to feel better than ever. Let's get started.

Chapter 1 – The Secret To Antibiotics

Whenever you go to the doctor, whether it's for an infection, a cough, an injury, or something similar, it doesn't take long before you are sent back out of the office with a prescription for antibiotics.

You are told to just take the pills at certain intervals, for a day, a couple days, or a few days, and whatever it is that bothers you is going to clear up. So, you do it.

And it works!

Within a few hours to a few days, whatever ailment you were facing begins to subside, and you are left feeling better than ever... or are you? Of course you may not have the ailment or illness anymore, but what is it exactly that you put into your body?

You can examine the bottle, skim over the ingredient list, and try to find what was actually in the medication, but the truth is, you just plain don't know. You see, many medications are actually produced in a lab, using synthetic substances.

These synthetic substances may make your illness go away, but are they doing you any good in return? Perhaps not.

Our bodies are designed to use the natural things in the world around us. Thousands of years ago, long before there were any science labs or synthetic substances, people were using natural remedies to care for the ailments they faced.

From cuts and burns to colds and fevers, plants were the main source of medication... and they worked.

There is overwhelming evidence of doctors and even surgeons spanning back over the centuries... long before anything remotely close to our modern medicine was in the world.

These doctors cared for their patients, and they were good at what they did... why? Because they knew what worked. They understood how to use herbal remedies for a variety of ailments, and how to create their own antibiotics right out of the plants they were growing in their gardens.

But, you may wonder, how did they know they needed antibiotics? They may not have called them such things, and they may not have realized that's what they were, but they did know how to use these plants and herbs to create their own medication, for anything they needed.

This all natural medication is far better than anything you will find in synthetic medication today, because it's real.

Even if you are getting good results with synthetic medication, you can't change the fact that it's not real, and your body has to deal with this. Your body wants to use real substances that grow naturally on the earth. It's how life itself is designed to be.

Let me show you how to use all natural antibiotics to get the same results synthetics provide.

Though it may seem hard to believe at first, you can treat yourself just as effectively with plants and herbs, without ever having to set foot inside a doctor's office.

This book is going to transform the way you view holistic medication, and save you thousands of dollars in doctor visits, prescriptions, and synthetic remedies that don't work.

Read on to discover how to manage your own holistic antibiotics. Once you have the right knowledge, you will never have to wait in line for another antibiotic prescription again. Go natural, and see how it works compared to the modern medicine.

The results are going to amaze you.

Chapter 2 – You're Doing It Wrong

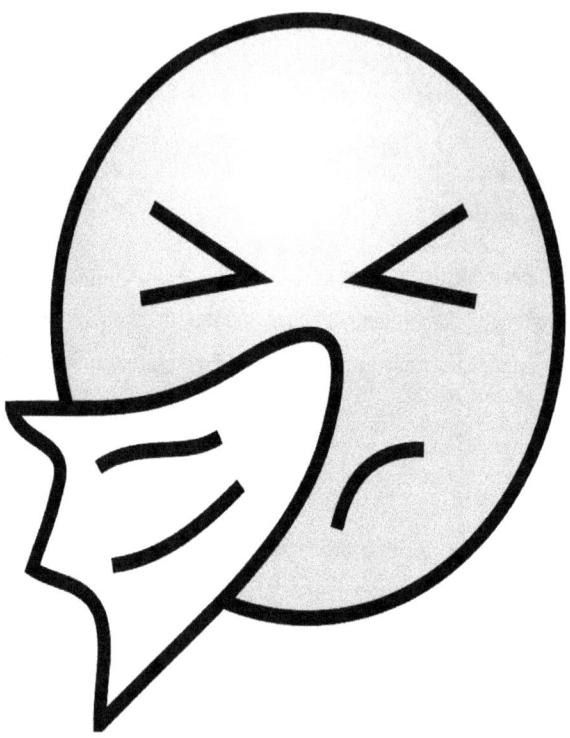

Right now, you wonder how I can be so certain holistic remedies are going to work. After all, you had a headache last year, you tried that old method your mother prescribed to you, and you ended up with a migraine.

Or perhaps you have watched your neighbor do countless detoxes and other natural remedies for countless things she has experienced, and you have never seen anything remarkable come of it. She always eventually heads to the doctor's office or comes back to the more modern way of handling things.

In our modern world, we are taught to criticize and be leery of any medication that didn't come out of a lab. Though you can purchase all natural supplements in the store, you are subjected to the implication they aren't as good... or as effective... as what you could get if you went synthetic.

The problem here isn't because supplements and all natural remedies aren't as good... it's the fact that many users don't know what they are doing. They assume these supplements and herbs are to be used as any other medication, and they simply try it once a day.

But they don't get the results they want. Though they take whatever it is as they would anything else, they are still left with the headache, the fever, or the risk of infection.

What they don't realize is that it's not the remedy that's the issue, it's the way they are using it.

Natural remedies aren't like synthetic. Yes, they are just as effective if not more so, but they have to be used properly in order to get the results you want. You can't just throw back some of the herbs and expect the same results, you have to put in the time and effort required.

Often when you use natural remedies, you have to use them in a tea or make a paste and apply the paste topically. This is going to be something you do more than once a day, in fact you may have to do it five or six times a day to get the results you want, but it's worth it.

When it comes to natural medication, you are giving your body the tools it needs to heal, but you have to also supply it with the right environment for that to happen. Stick with it, even when you don't see the results you want at first.

Be consistent with the use of the remedy, and be patient for the results. Though there are few cases when you have to go in and get your condition cared for by a doctor as soon as you can, more often than not you have time to treat it yourself.

In this modern world we live in, many people want instant results. If they can't have the illness completely healed within a couple of hours, they aren't going to give it a chance. But, the fact of the matter is, though synthetic medication may make you feel better quickly, it's not healing you any faster than natural remedies do.

Your body is going to take the time it needs to heal, whether you are using something all natural or not. Though one may feel as though using synthetics is working better than going all natural, it's not, and you are doing more harm to your body than you would be otherwise.

When it comes to using herbs to treat yourself or cure any illness you have, you have to approach the topic with an open mind. You can't just expect it all to work instantly, and you can't just assume anything is going to work for what you want it to.

There is going to be a fair share of trial and error before you get it just right, and you will have to be willing to go through this before you get the consistent results you are after. My best advice to keep this all to a minimum is to practice with your herbs when you feel great, so when you don't, you know what works and what doesn't.

When you are sick, you want relief, and the best way to get that is through using the herbal remedies that work. If you have already worked with them in the past, you know which ones these will be, but if not, you are going to put yourself through a lot of work just hoping for the best.

Of course, stand on my shoulders and along with those who have done the work before. There's a reason you find herbs on the lists of various remedies, and that's because others have done the work already.

But, everyone is different, and what works great for one may not work so well for another, so I encourage you to take the time to find what works for you before you go crazy with the remedies. Find the ones you enjoy, find the ones that work, and go with the ones you love.

This way, when you really do need them, you will have them right there and waiting for you. The key to success when using natural remedies is to know how to use them, and part of that knowledge means you have to put in the time in advance. There's so many ways you can use these, but you have to know what works, and what doesn't.

So let's get down to it. In the next chapter, we are going to start in on the herbs themselves.

Chapter 3 – The Remedies: Part 1

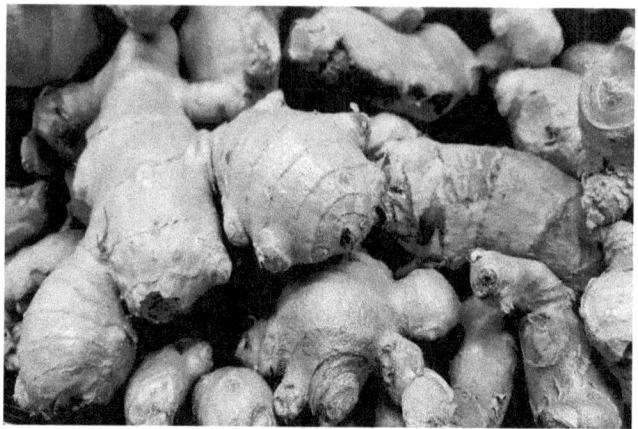

We have finally come to the part you have been waiting for... the herbs themselves. Of course, you can find all of these herbs online if you can't find them in store, so don't stress.

I have grouped them so you will find them easily, and be able to pick which herbs you want to use based on the illness you are dealing with. Again, feel free to mix and match as well as explore your options to find the one that works best for you.

There's no wrong way to do it, and you are more than welcome to blend a few herbs at a time to care for multiple symptoms. Think of it as creating your own customized tea made especially for you.

Things could not get better.

These herbs and holistic remedies are a blend of spices, herbs, and roots. You can use multiple parts of a plant to get the results you want, and you may even get to use multiple parts of the same plant if you do your research.

Make sure you know which parts of the plant are edible, and what you can use before you do, just because you can eat one part doesn't always mean you can eat another, and when it comes to herbs, you can never be too careful.

Common colds and ailments
Elder flowers
Ginger root
Echinacea
Umcka
Astralagus
Black pepper
Basil

Crushing the herbs and wrapping them in cloth is an easy way to make a tea, or if you can break them into smaller pieces, but not fully crush them, place them in a tea ball to steep for a while.

I find the best way to use these kinds of remedies is to steep them in water for a few minutes, then drink the tea. Repeat this for as many times as needed, or every couple of hours. When you are using herbal remedies, it's still possible to overdo it, but it's going to take a lot more to do that than it does with the synthetics, so don't worry.

Another option for use is to cruse these and blend them with some unscented body lotion of your choice, and to massage them into the affected areas. If you don't have body lotion on hand, try petroleum jelly, as this works well, too.

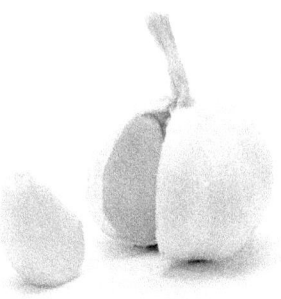

Infection care and infection prevention
Garlic
Cayenne
Cinnamon
Oregon grape root
Calendula

Crushing the herbs and wrapping them in cloth is an easy way to make a tea, or if you can break them into smaller pieces, but not fully crush them, place them in a tea ball to steep for a while.

I find the best way to use these kinds of remedies is to steep them in water for a few minutes, then drink the tea. Repeat this for as many times as needed, or every couple of hours. When you are using herbal remedies, it's still possible to overdo it, but it's going to take a lot more to do that than it does with the synthetics, so don't worry.

Another option for use is to cruse these and blend them with some unscented body lotion of your choice, and to massage them into the affected areas. If you don't have body lotion on hand, try petroleum jelly, as this works well, too.

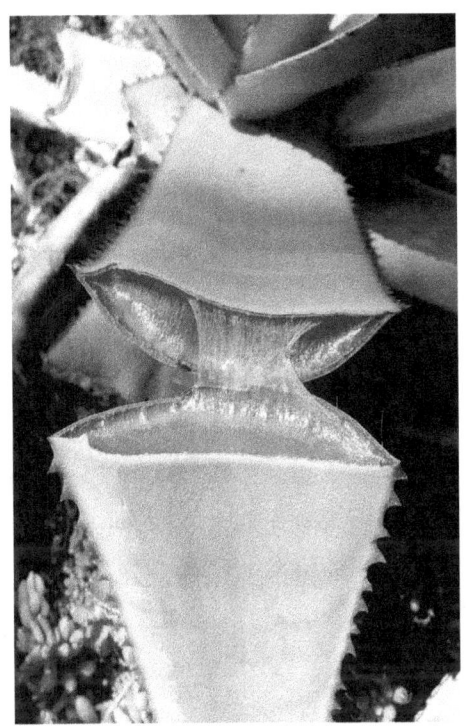

Minor scrapes and cuts

Balm of Gilead

Barberry root

Chickweed

Aloe leaves

Comfrey leaves

Crushing the herbs and wrapping them in cloth is an easy way to make a tea, or if you can break them into smaller pieces, but not fully crush them, place them in a tea ball to steep for a while.

I find the best way to use these kinds of remedies is to steep them in water for a few minutes, then drink the tea. Repeat this for as many times as needed, or every couple of hours. When you are using herbal remedies, it's still possible to overdo it, but it's going to take a lot more to do that than it does with the synthetics, so don't worry.

Though it seems unlikely, you can actually use teas to stave off infection when you have been injured. Think of it as the same idea of taking a round of antibiotics orally, even though you have cut yourself or experienced a similar ailment. Do what works for you, and what makes you feel best.

Another option for use is to cruse these and blend them with some unscented body lotion of your choice, and to massage them into the affected areas. If you don't have body lotion on hand, try petroleum jelly, as this works well, too.

When it comes to these herbs, you can use them for the symptoms I have recommended, or you can mix and match to get greater use out of them. As I said, you can create a tonic with more than one herb at a time, or you can stick with the one you want.

But, if you are dealing with a cold and a fever both, you may want to adjust the herbs you are using. If, however, you are only dealing with one thing in particular, you may want to adjust the herbs you are using based on what you are feeling. The greatest benefit you will get from using your own herbs is the freedom to use them as you want, when you want.

Explore your options and the results, and discover what you want to do. You can learn the right ways to use them from me, but you are the only one who can tell you if they are the herbs you want to use or not.

Don't be afraid of your herbs, get out there and explore all the things you can do with them! You never know what you can do until you try.

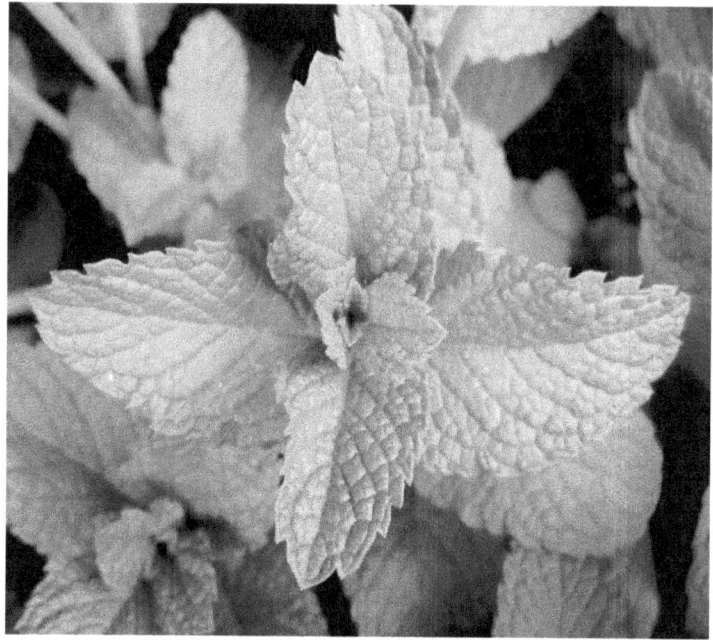

You've made it through the first list of plants and herbs, but that's only half. Here are the rest of the holistic antibiotics you should keep on hand for any ailment you may face.

Big or small, you will be happy you have them on hand.

For headaches

Peppermint

Spearmint

Passion flower

White willow bark

Lemon mint

Black cohosh

Crushing the herbs and wrapping them in cloth is an easy way to make a tea, or if you can break them into smaller pieces, but not fully crush them, place them in a tea ball to steep for a while.

I find the best way to use these kinds of remedies is to steep them in water for a few minutes, then drink the tea. Repeat this for as many times as needed, or every couple of hours. When you are using herbal remedies, it's still possible to overdo it, but it's going to take a lot more to do that than it does with the synthetics, so don't worry.

Another option for use is to cruse these and blend them with some unscented body lotion of your choice, and to massage them into the affected areas. If you don't have body lotion on hand, try petroleum jelly, as this works well, too.

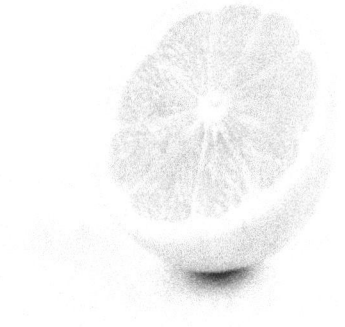

For stomach aches

Fennel seed

Lemon

Chamomile

Dandelion

Black licorice

Lavender

Crushing the herbs and wrapping them in cloth is an easy way to make a tea, or if you can break them into smaller pieces, but not fully crush them, place them in a tea ball to steep for a while.

I find the best way to use these kinds of remedies is to steep them in water for a few minutes, then drink the tea. Repeat this for as many times as needed, or every couple of hours. When you are using herbal remedies, it's still possible to overdo it, but it's going to take a lot more to do that than it does with the synthetics, so don't worry.

Another option for use is to cruse these and blend them with some unscented body lotion of your choice, and to massage them into the affected areas. If you don't have body lotion on hand, try petroleum jelly, as this works well, too.

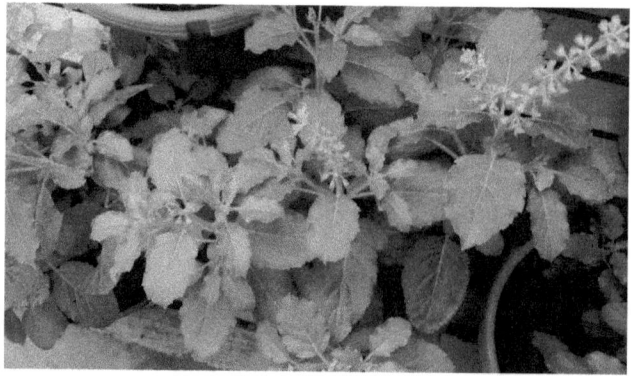

Body aches and pains

St John's wort

Kava kava

Ginseng

Valerian root

Turmeric

Holy basil

Crushing the herbs and wrapping them in cloth is an easy way to make a tea, or if you can break them into smaller pieces, but not fully crush them, place them in a tea ball to steep for a while.

I find the best way to use these kinds of remedies is to steep them in water for a few minutes, then drink the tea. Repeat this for as many times as needed, or every couple of hours. When you are using herbal remedies, it's still possible to overdo it, but it's going to take a lot more to do that than it does with the synthetics, so don't worry.

Another option for use is to cruse these and blend them with some unscented body lotion of your choice, and to massage them into the affected areas. If you don't have body lotion on hand, try petroleum jelly, as this works well, too.

Regardless of the herb you choose, make sure you do your research on the herb if you are taking any medication.

As I have said, you don't have to stress too much about overdosing on the herbs in and of themselves. Yes, it is possible, but it's not likely, especially if you are using them medicinally and not abusing them.

However, you do need to remember that these are herbs, and they are powerful. This means if you are using any other kind of medication, these could potentially make your medication work differently. If you have ever noticed that there are warnings on the sides of medication which ask if you are taking any supplements, this is why.

You don't have to be afraid of the herbs, but you do want to be aware of what you are putting into your body before you do it. If you are in doubt, talk to your doctor before you begin any of the herbal treatments.

He may want to encourage you to use synthetics for his own reasons, but that's fine. Simply ask him if you can use herbs with the medication you are taking, if he doesn't recommend it, see if there is some other medication you can switch to that does allow it.

At the end of the day, it never hurts to ask.

Chapter 5 – Home Grown Solutions

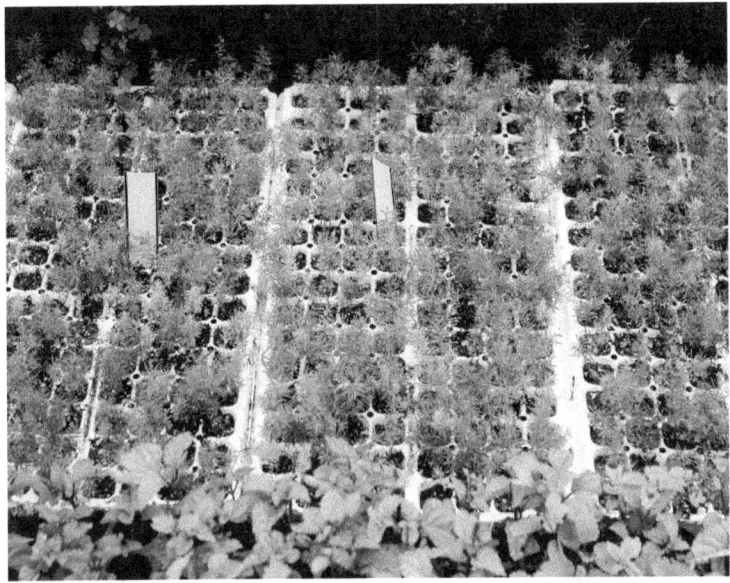

Knowing which kinds of herbs to grow is exciting, and knowing how to use those herbs properly is even more exciting, but nothing is as exciting as when you learn how you can grow these herbs in your own home, and maintain a constant supply of them to your family whenever you need.

As you already know, many of the starter plants or the seeds to these plants can be purchased locally or online if you aren't able to source them, and many of them can be purchased relatively inexpensively, especially when you compare them to the synthetic medication you have been purchasing before now.

However, purchasing the starter plants or the seeds is just part of the battle. If you want to be successful in growing your own herbs, you need to know how to grow them, and set up the right environment for them to grow.

This is going to require just the basics in your house, and you will be set to start almost immediately.

First, decide which herbs you want to grow, and plan accordingly

It's not going to take you long before you realize that these herbs require different settings to be able to grow effectively. There are some that need a lot of light, there are others that only need a little. Then there are more that have to have partial sunlight in order to grow at all.

You are going to find some that can grow nearly everywhere, then others that require specific temperatures and daylight hours in the day. You will have to pick and choose which herbs can grow in the same conditions, and which ones require special treatment.

If you are going to dive in with both feet, simply set up more than one place in the house for your plants, but if you are going to cater to only a few that can be grown in the same areas, then you only need to prepare a single place in your house for the project.

Either way, take the time to get it all set up and working before you bring in the plants, so they have a better chance of survival. The first few days are always the hardest on any new plants, even if you are planting them from seeds.

Give them time to settle in and take root, and gently keep water on them through this time. Don't slosh water on them, simply sprinkle a few drops here and there to ensure they are getting the moisture they need, but not drowning or getting uprooted.

It takes some time to get used to the process, but with a few days of trial and error, you will have it down. Work with a few different kinds of plants, especially if you can get the same results from using them, and discover the kinds you like the best.

Once you find your favorites to grow, you won't have an issue at all keeping them alive. This is going to allow you to keep that steady flow on hand no matter what time of year it is, or how often you need to use them.

When it comes to growing your own plants for herbal remedies, or using herbs as remedies for that matter, you are going to need to go through the trial and error period. They are going to work, but you have to do your part to find what works best for you.

With time, you will learn the ones that grow well, and how to use them. Then, nothing is going to stand in your way.

Here's to good health.

Conclusion

There you have it, everything you need to know about herbal remedies, and how you can use them to treat virtually any illness you face. I know you are used to living in a world where people tell you to run to the doctor every time you sneeze, but the fact of the matter is, you can really heal yourself with the right methods, quickly and easily.

I hope this book was able to inspire you to get on those methods, and that you are starting your own growing practice right now. All it takes is some pots and some soil, along with your preferred seeds, and you are set. There's no end to the ways you can make your own planters, and the plants you grow are virtually unlimited as well.

Use the list of plants in this book and find the ones that work best for you, or branch out and learn even more that you can use for herbal remedies. There's no way you can do it wrong, and when you are growing your own, you know without a doubt you are in control.

I want this book to show you just how easy it is for you to grow and use your own natural antibiotics, and I want this book to get you out of the doctor's office and back on your feet where you belong.

There's so many different ways you can use your remedies in your day, and once you discover just how easy it is, you will never want to go back. I want this book to be inspiring, and I want you to feel inspired to make the change you need to make.

There's no sense in putting those synthetic substances in your body any longer, and with the knowledge this book provides, you don't have to. Let me show you a whole new way of doing things, and how you can start growing... and using your very own herbal antibiotics today.

As you saw in this book, there are times when you need to do things that are unconventional, or downright different than what you have always done, and that's ok. With this book, I want to open your mind in more ways than one, and show you that you can experience modern medicine in a whole new way.

Safe, effective, and inexpensive, you will wonder why more people don't try herbal remedies for their needs.

No more stress, no more doctor's offices, and no more worries. You really can tend to all these things yourself, starting now.

www.ingramcontent.com/pod-product-compliance
Lightning Source LLC
Chambersburg PA
CBHW072101280526
45788CB00006B/2350